The

Chocolate Chip Cookie, Ice Cream, Cake, Brownie, and Pie Diet

(A Weight Stabilization Concept)

by

George Deeb

Published by

Artistions Expressic LLC

Business inquiries - artistionsexpressic@earthlink.net

Contents

Section 5

Section 6

Section 7

Section 8

ADDENDUM

What This Book Is About

This book is **NOT** about a **weight LOSS** program.

It **IS** about a **weight STABILIZATION** concept.

This book does **NOT** have **RECIPES** to follow.

This book is **NOT** a **joke**. It is about a very serious health problem happening in today's modern society, around the world, where lifestyles have gotten less physical and more sedate. Where most working age adults spend 8 hours or more, every week day (and some even on the weekends) in a mostly stationary and almost inactive position.

Section 2

1

Who this book IS FOR

If you put weight on easily, while eating seemingly small amounts of food when compared to other people – you should read this book.

If you have trouble controlling the ups and downs of your weight, and it always seems to mostly go up – you should read this book.

If you have had a life-long/years-long battle with controlling your weight – you should read this book.

If you have a weight problem, and you believe it is because you have a "slow metabolism" – you should read this book.

If you get most of your food and snacks in a processed and packaged form, and you have trouble controlling your weight – you should read this book.

If you have gone from a physically active life style to a more inactive one, and you were used to eating anything you wanted, but now find your weight is constantly increasing – you should read this book.

If, like myself, you can lose weight normally when on a weight loss program (diet), then gain it back at a seemingly fast rate when you stop the weight loss program – you should read this book.

If your weight is at an "acceptable" level, but you have to constantly be careful of what you eat – you should read this book

If you are leaving home, where real food was made for you, and going out on your own to end up eating processed, packaged food because it is easy and quick – you should read this book.

If most of the food you eat is prepackaged, processed foods – you DEFINITELY should read this book.

For simplicity's sake, in this book I will refer to this **weight stabilization concept** interchangeably as a "diet" or a "concept". This **weight stabilization** concept does not require you to buy any special foods, buy any special supplements, or buy anything you can't get at your local grocery. Nor does it restrict your food intake, or follow any special program. If you follow this concept, and do not habitually over-eat, you should be able to continue eating the way you like. In most cases, this concept does not cost you any more money than what you are already spending on food.

Is this dieting concept for me if I have a different kind of weight problem? – I don't have the answer to that question. This weight stabilization concept MAY help if you have a different kind of weight problem. You won't know until you try it. But first, you have to **understand it**. I will try to explain it the best way I can in this book.

2

Who and what this book IS NOT FOR

This book is not needed by everybody. However, this weight stabilization concept can only improve your health.

This book is not for losing weight, although you may lose some at a very slow rate. I have included, at the end of the book, some specific data showing how this stabilization concept has affected my weight (It's boring stuff, but will give you an idea of the concept's results – my own personal results).

This book is not for binge eating or binge dieting. If you follow my diet concept you may not want to, or feel you have to, do either of these anyway.

Section 3

1

How this concept came about

This whole thing started because of the lousy taste of commercially produced chocolate chip cookies (my personal addiction) found in retail markets today. Not only was the taste lousy, it was inconsistent (Poor quality control?). The same product (chocolate chip cookie) from the same manufacturer brand would rarely have the same taste and/or texture as a previous purchase (Just days or a week prior!). To make it even worse, sometimes it would just taste bad (Road trip for a store return, anyone?}. It didn't matter who the manufacturer/brand was (I've tried many), or whether it was a highly advertised, well known name brand, or a store brand (A lot of them probably come from the same plant/commercial-baking facility that is contracted to produce these products in your area – just a guess).

Let me start at the beginning. I am addicted to chocolate chip cookies. Have been ever since my early twenties. I don't know why, and I don't know how this started. I actually got cravings for them that overrode my conscious desire not to buy any more (in an attempt to try to stop my increasing weight). Any conscious control and will power to stay away from them disappeared from my mind once the craving manifested. For you, it may be something other than chocolate chip cookies that affect you in the same way.

For me, getting cookies had meant getting it from a store (Either a grocery market or "bakery" section of a market. More on bakeries later.). It is hard to say for certain (I am working on memory here), but it seems that many years ago, if you bought a name brand package of cookies and went back for another package at some later date, the taste and texture would be the same or close to the same. But, for the last decade or so (possibly longer), that no longer seemed to be the case. Whether this is due to a change in recipe, ingredients, production facility, manufacturing practices, a change in my taste buds, a change in something I am not aware of, or all of the above, I don't know. My guess is that it is an ingredient and quality control issue. Whatever the reason, it is the present reality. Quality control doesn't seem to exist anymore. Sometimes they taste like paste, and other times they taste like uncooked flour. Sometimes they will be relatively thick, and sometimes thin. Sometimes crispy and sometimes crunchy. Sometimes I can't tell what it is that they taste like, other than disappointing or just bad.

I also had a different problem with places that specialized in cookies and baked goods (Pick any well know chain store known for its baked treats). They all seemed to make their chocolate-chip cookies with too much sugar/sweetener (they seem to think that sweet is a flavor), or too much chocolate (What??? He's complaining about too much chocolate???). Bakery-chain bought choco-chip cookies seemed more like a chocolate bar with some cookie dough added in than a cookie with some chocolate chips added in.

Now, I don't doubt that kids and young adults might like it that way, and even that it might be good for retail sales. But my tastes have become more demanding and specific. To me, a chocolate chip cookie should be a cookie (a good tasting one) with chocolate chips that don't overpower everything else. A cookie from which I can taste the cookie and the chips separately. AND one that does not use sugar (or some sweetener) as a flavor ingredient (I am guessing that sweeteners must be very cheap in commercial quantities). To anyone in the cookie making industry that might read this book, let me educate you on one thing – sugar is NOT a flavoring (and certainly artificial sweeteners do not make anything taste good).

A couple of years ago I reached a point where I was no longer willing to put up with it. So I did one of the only logical things I could do to resolve the problem. My choices were to either find a local bakery (a real bakery that makes goods from scratch, using common ingredients) that made the treats I liked (No luck there. I don't have any real bakeries near me.), or to make them myself.

2

The way it <u>WAS</u> for me

When it comes to eating, I have lived what I would consider to be a fairly normal, city oriented modern day American style life. For most of my life, I acquired most of my food and snacks from a grocery store. Having a sweet tooth, and being someone who didn't know and (at that time) didn't desire to learn how to cook meant that most of my food was processed, prepackaged, or came from restaurants. A microwave was the only oven that I had any familiarity with, and its use was limited to re-heating. It is very tempting (especially with a busy schedule) to pull something out of the freezer, put it in the microwave, and be eating a few minutes later – quick and easy.

When I desired a cookie, I would go to the store and buy a package of cookies. While I was watching TV in the evening, I would open that package and start eating them. I would eat six to ten cookies before I had any sense of being satisfied. That usually led to two scenarios. ONE – I would leave what was left near me (within reach), and in ten or so minutes I would be grabbing for another cookie. If it was early enough in the evening, I might end up finishing that package. That's two dozen cookies in one evening. TWO – If I didn't finish the package, there might be three to six cookies left that evening. Guess what I would have with my morning coffee?

The next day came with the self-admonishment that I was being foolish and irresponsible, knowing that some time down the road I would have to be on a weight loss diet again. Resolving to myself that I would not buy any more cookies, I was determined to stick with the plan. That would last about two days, and then the memory of my resolution would completely vanish from my mind. It would start all over again. Seemed to be a never ending cycle.

3

The way it <u>IS</u> for me now

At present, I might eat two to four cookies in a day. This leaves me satisfied, and feeling full. Thoughts of having more are gone for the rest of the day. I know longer have to resolve not to eat any more cookies because <u>I intend to do just that</u>, while <u>not worrying anymore about gaining weight</u>. I may or may not eat any more. But if I decide to, I no longer have to worry about gaining weight from them. These are cookies that I bake in my own kitchen, and not commercially produced. Some days, I might not eat any cookies. That doesn't mean I haven't eaten any snacks, just not cookies (which are my primary craving). My cookies are made with sugar, butter, flour, salt, leavening, eggs, vanilla extract, and chocolate chips. This recipe does NOT include anything that I can't pronounce, and that isn't normally found in the average home kitchen.

Before I realized how to stabilize my weight (and what it was that was causing my weight gain), I would not dare to bring home a whole carrot cake, or cheesecake, or pie, or so many other things, because I knew that if it was inside the house I would end up eating it. Now, I don't give it any thought. The difference now is that I make my own cake, or pie, or other treat, WITH the intention of eating the whole thing. Today, I can do so and know that my weight will not increase.

When I was eating commercial cookies, it would take many of them before I felt satisfied, and that feeling only lasted for a short time before I would be eating more. Any energy that I felt from eating them was slow to appear, and would diminish quickly. I would soon feel physically weak and needing to eat again. Of course, my first thoughts of what to eat would be more of those commercially made cookies.

Now that I have dropped the commercially produced cookies, it takes less of them to fill me up, and the energy I feel can last for five hours or more (depending on my activity at the time). The most surprising thing I have noticed is that hours later, when I am feeling hungry again, I don't feel a lack of energy. If I am in the middle of something, I can push the hunger out of my mind and finish the project. I was not able to do that before. After being on my non-processed foods program for almost a couple of years now, that ability to ignore hunger pangs still surprises me.

4

Adding insult to injury

Have I mentioned that I had very bad eating habits? Most of the foods that I ate were processed in some way. Yes, it was very convenient to take something out of the freezer and place it in the microwave. Yes, it wasn't great tasting or had a good texture, but it wasn't that bad. Frozen foods have come a long way from the early days when they tasted like cardboard. And usually, it was quick and easy. For some foods, I had no concept of what it should taste like when made correctly.

5

What is meant by processed food?

I am not referring to mechanically processed food, as in grinding meat or grains. By the term "processed food" I mean CHEMICALLY processed food. The simplest (and maybe best) definition of a processed food is one that contains ingredients you wouldn't have in the average home kitchen, or that you can't pronounce. So, what am I talking about here. Below is a list of some of those ingredients from cake mixes:

Propylene Glycol (Isn't that used in anti-freeze?)
Mono- and Diesters of Fats and Fatty Acids
Mono- and Diglycerides
Sodium Stearoyl Lactylate
Sodium Aluminum Phosphate
Monocalcium Phosphate
Artificial Flavors (not specified)
Cellulose Gum (WHAT ???)
Xanthan Gum
Yellow 5 Lake
Red 40 Lake
Soy Lecithin

Sodium Caseinate

Bht

etc.

And here are some from commercially produced cookies:

Canola oil

Palm and palm kernel oil

High fructose corn syrup

Dextrose

Soy lecithin

Artificial flavor (not specified)

Caramel color (not specified)

Soybean oil

REDUCED IRON

THIAMINE MONONITRATE

hydrogenated palm kernel oil

sodium acid pyrophosphate

monocalcium phosphate

Here are some of the ingredients in Hostess Twinkies:

sorbic acid and potassium sorbate (to retain freshness)

cottonseed oil (when has cotton been considered a food item?)

mono and diglycerides

cellulose gum

sodium stearoyl lactylate

polysorbate 60

monocalcium phosphate

artificial flavor (what is it and where did it come from?)

yellow 5

red 40

According to the CVS Pharmacy web page (at the time of this writing in 2021), and in contrast to some of the above items, is the ingredients list in a Snickers candy bar:

MILK CHOCOLATE (SUGAR, COCOA BUTTER, CHOCOLATE, SKIM MILK, LACTOSE, MILKFAT, SOY LECITHIN, ARTIFICIAL FLAVOR), PEANUTS, CORN SYRUP, SUGAR, PALM OIL, SKIM MILK, SALT, EGG WHITES, ARTIFICIAL FLAVOR.

Wow! I almost know what all of those ingredients are. Maybe I should make a snickers bar part of my regular diet. But, don't forget that there might be ingredients that aren't separately listed on a product's label. Notice above all the ingredients they use to make the milk chocolate. Sometimes an ingredient just listed as a single item, such as "milk chocolate", without telling the consumer what is used to make it.

If you don't know what it is, stay away from it if possible. Even some ingredients that you do know are not good for this diet concept. Unfortunately, I don't know which ones all of them are. Now, not all strange or exotic sounding ingredients are bad. The problem is how to know which ones are bad for you. I am not a doctor, or a chemist. I don't have a lab or a research facility. I haven't run any large group testing. Your guess is as good as mine. The only way you and I can find out is to try something and see what the end result is. If your weight goes up, maybe it's an ingredient or product that you want to stay away from. I am not saying you should purchase some strange sounding additive, and swallow some. I am saying that if you see it in the ingredients list of something you ate, you know you have consumed some of it.
In the mean time, I can tell you one of the processed foods that I

stay away from (as I've said before) – commercially produced cookies (All of them that have chemicals in their ingredients list. Not just the chocolate chip that I am addicted to). By commercially produced, I mean the kind you find available in large quantities at retail stores. If there are stacks of packages of them on the shelves, they are commercially produced.

6

Strange stuff, or just strange names?

So why are these things with strange names put into our food? They are used for many reasons:

Some of the main ones are:
– They extend shelf life.
– Because they are cheaper than the natural ingredients they substitute for.
– They make the product softer, chewier, crispier, crunchier, more palatable (since the other chemical ingredients don't taste very good).
– They make the product look prettier (shinier, darker in color, lighter in color, a particular color, etc.).
– They give the product a desired texture.

As more people around the world turned to processed foods for their convenience (just like us), we have moved away from more natural (i.e. non-processed) foods made from individual ingredients, at home.

7

What in processed foods are bad for me?

I wish I had a list I could give you. The problem is that some people can eat any processed food they want and have no obvious ill effects. It is the people like you and I, the ones that are affected, who have to change our buying and eating habits. Some processed foods may not have any bad effect on you, while some will. The specific ill effect that I am focusing on in this book is body weight, which is often related to other physiological problems. That doesn't mean that just because it isn't obvious, there isn't anything bad going on. People who don't have weight issues with processed foods may have other things going on caused by these chemicals, and they just haven't made the connection between the two. Remember that we are talking about chemicals whose effects are slow acting in the amounts ingested, and can take a long period of time to show up. It's hard to make a connection to something that doesn't have an immediate effect.

8

Aren't processed foods necessary in today's world economy?

Today, we may have the convenience and availability of foods brought in from around the world, in our local grocery store. Some of these items are processed foods. Luckily, a lot of them are not. Preserving food by canning, or bottling is not the same as being chemically processed. Avoiding processed foods does not limit our choices by much (unless you are addicted to some particular manufactured product).

Throughout the world, today, there are people starving. They sometimes are lucky to get one scant meal a day. For some of us, that is hard to imagine. Being overweight is the last thing these people have to worry about. Chemical preservatives that give a longer shelf life to food products can be an important and even necessary way to process foods that will provide needed nutrition for starving people. The use of these chemicals can serve a useful purpose, especially in places without electricity or refrigeration. It isn't that these chemicals are a bad thing. It is that for some people, these chemicals can have an unwanted physiological effect.

Section 4

1

Who and what I am, and am not

I am a 68 inch tall male who's weight has been over 180 pounds for so long that I can't remember when I got there. My physical activity level is sedate-moderate, and varies with the seasons. Various "normal" body height and weight charts indicate that my ideal weight should be 125 to 158 pounds. I'd be very happy to see 158 again (Who am I kidding? I'd be very happy to see 170 again). With the occasional diet I would go on, I have seen my weight drop to 165. The problem is that my body weight would climb again when I went off the diet. And when I say climb, I mean climb rapidly. I could see the weight increasing on a **weekly** basis. This would happen even while I was trying to be careful about what and how much I ate.

In my opinion, being on a diet plan for the rest of your life is not a good way to live. I don't believe I could ever do that, anyway (Could anyone?). What bothered me the most was that no matter how much or how little I ate, my weight would increase. Something didn't make sense. Of course, as I now know, I was too blind to see what was in front of me. I was eating the only way I knew how. It wasn't the amount of food that was causing my problem. It was the type of food. And I'm not talking about salad versus dessert.

2

But I am still overweight. What do I do about that?

I have tried several of the commercial pre-packaged food type diets available, and for myself they worked well. There are also doctor monitored diets for those with a condition that requires professional supervision. If weight loss is needed, then a weight loss type of diet will be necessary to lose the pounds.

What happens after you have reached your weight goal, and it's time to end the diet? Usually, one of two things happen. Some people can successfully keep the weight off (or so I have heard. I don't personally know anyone who has done this.), while others end up watching their weight climb back up, and they can see it happen almost on a daily basis. If you gained just two pounds a month, you would be twenty-four pounds heavier by the end of a year. Who wants to be on, or is able to maintain, a diet for the rest of their lives? I know I couldn't do that. That was the situation I was in. No matter how successful my weight loss dieting was, it seemed beyond my control to keep the excess weight off. What I needed, and didn't know at the time, was a weight STABILIZATION plan. That was something I had never heard of before. In a time when we are surrounded with processed foods, and no one making it clear that they pose this type of potential problem, how was I (or anyone else) to know.

We often hear about how high sugar or fat content foods are bad for our health, and that they will make you fat. That was a simple message. What the message failed to take into account was all of the chemicals and substitute fats (trans fats) in our foods today. What wasn't explained was why some people were affected while others seemed immune. No one seemed to focus on or explain why that was. Maybe because the health professionals weren't aware of the metabolic connection to the additives in the foods that are all around us. Trans fats are now considered bad for your health, and I believe that is backed up with actual medical data. If there is any such data on why chemical additives cause weight increase I haven't been able to find it.

3

How do I check my weight results

Your body weight changes constantly. You can weigh yourself in the morning, and in the evening of the same day, and get different readings. The best way that I have found to see what is happening with my weight is to measure it once a week, on the same day and at about the same time, naked.

I weigh myself on Saturday mornings, right after I wake up, before I have had anything to eat. There is nothing special about Saturday, or the morning. It is just convenient for me. I recommend you use a scale with a digital readout, if possible. If you don't have a digital scale, but have an analog one, use what you have. Just be aware that analog scale readings might vary slightly due to inherent inaccuracies built into the mechanical system, unless it is a good quality scale (which a lot of home scales are not). This error seems to be less with the digital scales.

Also, be aware that your reading from one week to another is not important. What is important is the long term trend of your weight. That said, four to five weeks (four to five measurements as outlined above) should be enough to give you a reliable indication of what is happening with your weight.

Also important is to **use the same scale** for your readings. You can't weigh yourself with your home scale one week, and be at your friend's house using their scale the next, while expecting a reliable trend. There are always differences between non-calibrated scales, which most home scales are. To get a reliable trend, you have to take consistent readings – same day each week, at about the same time, using the same scale.

4

How soon will I see results

The effect of this concept begins immediately after you eliminate the processed foods from your diet. As soon as you eliminate these chemicals from your diet you will be having an effect on your weight. As to when you will actually see results, you have to remember that you will be weighing yourself only once a week, and that you are looking for a trend. That trend may not be seen clearly until the end of the first month.

If you want, you can weigh yourself more often, but the same rules will apply. If you want to weigh yourself every Saturday morning and every Wednesday evening, you can do that. More than likely you will see a difference of several pounds between the two readings. That is not important. What is important is the trend for every Saturday, and the trend for every Wednesday. I am not sure doing this on different days will be helpful in any way, but if it makes you happy then do it.

If you don't see your weight stabilizing after a month, it probably means that either something else is affecting you and you may need to follow a weight loss program, or that you haven't eliminated the chemicals from your diet and you need to look closer at the ingredients of what you are eating. The best way to be sure you are following the stabilization concept correctly is to make your own food (or have someone you know make it for you) with ingredients that you know.

5

Calories In – Calories Used

This weight stabilization concept is not a magic bullet (although sometimes it seems like it is). It can't change the fact that if you take in more calories than your body uses, you will gain weight. What it changes is the ability of your body to utilize the food that you eat, instead of creating fat to lock away chemicals it doesn't know how to process. Think about this – you just ate a meal, made with chemically processed foods. You are one of the people whose body can't utilize or immediately eliminate these chemicals. You body does the only other thing it can do – lock the chemical away in body fat. Body fat equates to energy that is derived from the food you ate. Since some of that energy is now stored away, that meal has supplied you with less usable energy than it should have. Since less energy is available, you will need more energy sooner than if your body could have utilized all the energy available in the meal. That means you will feel hungry again sooner than you should have, and that means you will eat more often.

Good eating habits are still important. If your idea of a good meal is to eat until your stomach is about to burst, then this concept will not help you control your weight. I can tell you from personal experience following this system, that I have had less cravings, as well as less desire to eat as often or as much, as I had before following the concept.

6

Will I lose weight?

It is possible. I have. But, the weight loss will be very small and very slow. Let me rephrase that – the weight loss will be **VERY** slow. Again from personal experience, I have had a half pound of weight loss in five to six weeks. The reason I know that this was true weight loss is that my weight held or dropped in the following weeks. As of this writing, it continues to do so. Lately, I have been experimenting (pushing the limits) with how much extra desserts I can eat and still hold my weight (It's a very tasty experiment). I have been amazed at the results. I have come to an end of the experiment, and will start to eat more normally now. This should result in some loss of weight, but I do not expect it to be very much or very fast. If your goal is to lose weight in a more substantial manner, you should go on a weight LOSS program. Then, after losing the weight, you can follow this weight stabilization concept. I have no doubt at all that you will enjoy following this weight stabilization concept MUCH more than the weight loss diet.

Section 5

1

Are processed foods bad for me?

According to the 2020 report published in the Medical News Today newsletter:

"chemically processed foods, also called ultra-processed foods, tend to be high in <u>sugar</u>, artificial ingredients, <u>refined carbohydrates</u>, and <u>trans fats</u>. Because of this, they are a major contributor to <u>obesity</u> and illness around the world."

"In recent decades, ultra-processed food intake has increased dramatically worldwide. These foods now account for **25–60% of a person's daily energy intake throughout much of the world."** (The bold is my emphasis)

Personally, I know this used to be true for myself (and maybe even more than 60% in my case). You can read the report for yourself at https://www.medicalnewstoday.com/articles/318630. It is not a very long article, and is very enlightening. The problem with the above statements is that they do not explain how or why these foods are bad for you. Most people reading them will think the obvious – that eating a lot of sugar, carbs, and trans-fats will, of course, put weight on you. I do not believe it is that simple. I will explain what I think is happening in a later section.

2

What about eating at restaurants

There is no problem with restaurant dining, if the restaurant makes its food they way you would make it at home. I would hate to have to give up my weekend brunches at my favorite restaurant. But, there are restaurants that use a lot of processed foods in their kitchens, and those should be avoided if identified. Usually, these are places that use pre-packaged, pre-cooked foods that just have to be heated up before they serve it to you. I find less of these places around these days, but that may not be the situation where you are at. Sometimes it's obvious that they are doing that, and sometimes not so easy to determine. Also, just because something is frozen doesn't mean it has chemical preservatives in it. On the other hand, some frozen foods do use chemical preservatives. Don't change your normal routines until you determine that an establishment has foods with additives in it that adversely affect you.

3

So, what is going on here

To put it simply, your body has a limited number of ways it can utilize what you ingest. The physiological processes involved with digestion are complex, but what we are interested in is the overall end result. When you eat or drink something, your body can do one of the following with it:

1) Utilize it immediately or in a short period of time
2) Store it for later use
3) Eliminate it
4) A combination of the above

The problem occurs when you ingest something that your body was not intended to utilize or doesn't know how to utilize, such as a synthetic product or an unnatural chemical additive. When that happens, the above end results change to the following because the additive can't be utilized. Your body:

1) Can't utilize it immediately, so it is stored (put aside and locked away, usually in body fat)
2) Can't utilize it at all, so it is kept stored, making it difficult for the body fat that is storing it to be utilized
3) Will eliminate it, if possible
4) Will convert it to something that may be harmful to your health, in the long or short term
5) Will have an adverse physiological response, in the long or short term
6) Will suffer internal system (organ) damage, that may occur in the long or short term (such as Cirrhosis of the liver caused by ingestion of alcohol over a long period of time)
7) Will have some of its normal processes hindered or impaired
8) Will experience a combination of the above

Some of the above reactions can be serious, but are not in the scope of this book. We are interested in those affecting body weight. That is the hypothesis of this weight stabilization concept. Items 1, 2, 4, 5, and 7 above are mainly what we are concerned with (although the others certainly do not help in keeping you healthy).

Here is my theory: The body weight of some people is affected adversely by the chemical additives in processed foods, more so than other people. Within the scope of this book, those people tend to accumulate body fat at an abnormally faster rate, due to the adverse effect of additives in processed foods. This abnormal increase in body fat happens because the body doesn't know what to do with the strange chemicals that were ingested, or the chemicals are directly stimulating an increase in body fat. The fat is used to lock away the chemicals, or hold them at bay because of trouble eliminating them from the body. Some people are also unable to utilize that stored fat without a drastic change in diet. Hence, they must follow a weight loss diet to get rid of the weight. But, when they go off the weight loss diet they experience (suffer?) the unreasonably rapid weight gain again. This is due to their bodies not knowing what to do with the chemicals that are being ingested, or being forced to do something abnormal by these chemicals.

Section 6

1

Where I've come from to where I am now

Throughout this book, I have often referenced sweets, snacks, treats, or whatever you want to call them, as my problem foods. My diet before also included in large part other processed foods (not snacks or sweets) because they were convenient to keep in the freezer, ready to just be warmed up and eaten. It was convenient, quick, and easy. So I really had two problem areas to contend with. At present, I avoid all of those as much as possible. I now do most of my cooking from scratch whenever possible (Well worth it as I enjoy eating the delicious results). My diet is more diverse, delicious, and healthy (I am eating more vegetables these days, also), and my culinary skills have improved tremendously. I like trying new recipes, and exploring different cuisines. I am still a sweets addict, and eat a lot of sweets and desserts, but now it is <u>without the weight gain</u>. I used to think I had a slow metabolism because of a relatively sedate life style, but now find my metabolism can handle what used to be too much for it before.

Let me try to push that point home. Today, following this weight stabilization concept, I am eating more food, and more sweets and treats than I did before (when I was seemingly always fighting my weight gain). I am doing this without my weight increasing!

At the end of this book, I have included a spreadsheet and chart of my weight over several months. In the spreadsheet is a list of the extra treats and sweets that I have eaten each week. Eating these extras is in addition to eating my regular meals and my everyday chocolate chip cookies that I keep on hand 24x7. This is not a complete list, as there were other snacks as well (a handful of chocolate chips here, some toasted pecans there, etc.). So, I am eating regular meals as well as more sweets than I used to eat when I was gaining weight, **while maintaining the same weight**. It may sound like I am repeating myself, but that's because I am trying to get the message across to you as best as I can.

2

Does this mean I have to make

all my meals myself

Unless you have a personal chef or can afford to eat out at a restaurant all the time, then yes it does. What I do is cook a couple of different dishes that serves 4 to 6, and eat them throughout the week, alternating them for variety, while throwing in the occasional restaurant pizza, and going out for breakfast now and then. I like to try something new once a week for added variety. I found that I like trying new recipes. Sometimes I keep it simple, and sometimes I make something more challenging to cook. How you want to handle it is up to you. There are several companies that will ship you premeasured ingredients packages for meals that you cook at home, so this would at least make it a little easier and save you some time. Don't worry – I understand they send instructions with each package. I have never used them, but my understanding is that they send real ingredients, and not processed food packs.

3

Does this mean I have to go organic

Going organic in your food purchases is not a bad idea. Personally, I haven't gone to that extreme. I do make sure that any produce I buy is washed well before I use it, so that I get the chemicals on the outside washed off. This would include pesticide residue, dirt, coatings, etc., and doesn't really fit into the same category as the chemicals used in processed foods, as far as I know.

4

People are people are people! Aren't they?

Everybody is physiologically different. Even within the same close family there are differences among the members. People in large families are usually aware of this because having so many persons in one place makes the differences more obvious. Sometimes the physiological differences are subtle and small. Sometimes they are drastic and large.

My brother-in-law had a friend who was proverbially skinny as a rail. He could pack away a whole casserole in one sitting. He could eat like that regularly and would not gain any weight. It's a good thing for him that he worked at a grocery store, where he got his food at a discount price. He was an obvious example of being physiologically different than so many of us.

We are also different in the way we live our lives. Some people are active all the time, and some have a more sedate life style. In today's world, more and more people are going to the sedate life because of our jobs. Modern day jobs have a lot of us sitting at a desk all day, which is not good for several reasons. With the invention of the computer, the situation got worse. If we focus only on the calories burned during the day, it is easy to see why our body weight tends to keep increasing. Having some form of physical activity as part of our lives is more important than ever before.

It doesn't matter if it is a weight loss program or a weight stabilization concept, it still comes down to calories taken in versus calories used up. We can't get away from that equation. Some of us use more calories than others, while doing the same activity. We are all different in some ways.

5

How sure are you that this will work for other people?

It may be that I am the only person, in a world of almost 8 billion people, that this works for. I would doubt it, but I have no way of knowing it as a fact, as of this writing. Or, you and I might be the only two people it works for. Or maybe, there is a whole bunch of people this concept will work for. If you fall into one of the problem categories described at the beginning of this book, wouldn't it be worth a try to find out if it will work for you?

6

What is the conclusion

I will let you draw your own conclusion, so here are the facts as they pertain to me. These days, I am eating more food (quantity and variety), as well as more sweets and treats (more calories) than I have ever eaten before when I was seeing my weight climb steadily. My weight now is staying at one place. It is both scary and exciting to get on the scale once a week, thinking that this can't be real. It is scary because I know all the treats I have eaten that week. It is exciting to see my weight holding steady. I think to myself that it can't be happening with all that I am eating. But it is real. It is happening to me.

Think about it. In one week, besides my regular meals, and however many cookies I ate, and some miscellaneous snacks I didn't keep track of, I also ate a whole cheesecake – or maybe it was whole loaf of banana bread – or a whole pie – or 8 to 10 chocolate covered peanut butter bars (or was it 16 of them?) – or a dish of brownies (all the aforementioned is true, by the way), and when I weigh myself Saturday morning my weight is still the same plus or minus a half pound. The trend over time averages out to being flat or going down.

It got to a point where I was wondering if my scale was broken. So, I picked up a 25 pound dumbbell, and the scale showed 25 pounds more. I did the same with a 10 pound dumbbell and again my scale read correctly. The strangest part is that I am still having trouble believing what is happening. It is still so new to me.

During another week, when I knew I had stuffed my face more than usual as well as eating an untested processed food (a different brand of ice cream with a different ingredients list), my weight went up 2.8 pounds. It was a shock, but not a surprise (I had eaten a LOT that week). The following week, after eating normally again, my weight dropped 1.8 of those new pounds. Three weeks later I was back where I had started from. There seems to be a regulating as well as a stabilizing effect occurring.

My only regret is that I didn't discover this when I was at a lower weight. Maybe in the future I will decide to go on a weight loss diet again to get my weight down, and then follow my weight stabilization concept to keep it there.

I am not advocating that someone live on cookies, cakes, and pies. I have no doubt that some people who read this book will have eating habits as bad as mine were. But, to be able to enjoy these treats without seeing my weight climb with almost every bite is not only a physical boon, but a psychological one as well. There is some peace of mind gained when you don't have to always be thinking about everything you are eating.

Section 7

1

Phthalates (Plastics)

Do you know how much plasticizer you are ingesting?

Do you know those pliable, milky-looking plastic bottles that milk, water, and other beverages are sold in? You probably already buy something in one of those bottles. If you buy water in one of those bottles, you will notice an obvious bad taste to it. That's the plasticizer leaching into the water (or other liquid). To put it bluntly, that stuff is **BAD** for you. I have always hated that taste (luckily for me), and from early on in the bottled water rage I stopped buying any products in that type of plastic. That is not to say that the problem isn't present with other plastics, but it is more obvious with that kind of container when it is used to package food. If you buy milk in those containers, you are feeding that chemical to yourself and your family. This is a scary thought when you think of exposing growing children to this chemical.

In a 2014 Q&A article from the Yale School of Medicine, titled "Is It Safe? Plasticizers in Personal Products" by Gary Ginsberg, PH.D., the question is asked:

Question – "I have heard that there are plasticizers in body lotion, deodorant and perfume. Is this true? If so, what are they doing there and will it harm me to wear these products on my skin?"

Doctor Ginsberg's answer is very frightening.

Answer – "This is a very important topic. People worry about toxic chemicals in all sorts of places, from cleaning products to couch cushions. Not that those aren't important, but probably the greatest exposure is from what you wear on your skin all day. This kind of intimate contact gives chemicals the chance to be absorbed into the body. The plasticizers that you are referring to are called phthalates. Although they have been banned from children's toys, they are in many personal care products. Their purpose is to help dissolve the fragrances in the product and then fix them to your skin. On average, women use 12 personal care products per day and men use about half that many. Most of these products contain fragrance and thus phthalates. These plasticizers are not known to damage the skin, **but once absorbed can disrupt the natural hormones, inhibiting testosterone and enhancing estrogen. Associations have been seen between phthalate exposure and breast cancer in women and low fertility in men** (see new research at: http://ens-newswire.com/2014/03/05/high-phthalate-levels-in-males-delays-pregnancy-in-partners/). **Phthalates cross the placenta and have been associated with improper development of baby boys.** While phthalates **do not have to be on the label** they are usually present with fragrance, an ingredient that is on the label. Essential oils make for pleasing scents and are usually phthalate-free. Look for essential oils rather than "fragrance" on the label to move beyond plasticized products for your skin."

The words in bold type are my emphasis. Please read those sentences again, especially the one that says "**Phthalates cross the placenta and have been associated with improper development of baby boys.**" The link listed in the answer is no longer valid. The corrected link is https://www.nih.gov/news-events/news-releases/high-plasticizer-levels-males-linked-delayed-pregnancy-female-partners and is from the National Institutes of Health.

If plasticizers "**can disrupt the natural hormones, inhibiting testosterone and enhancing estrogen**", I have to wonder what effect they have on body weight. I don't know exactly which chemical is being leached from those bottles, but why would anyone want to ingest an industrial chemical in any food item? Especially when you don't know what effect it is having on your body.

Pregnant women, especially, should be concerned about this. The statement "**Phthalates cross the placenta and have been associated with improper development of baby boys.**" means that developing girls are also exposed to the chemical. No known association to the developing female fetus is mentioned, but that only means that they haven't identified one yet.

What kind of birth defects will it cause, and how subtle will they be at first? What problems will it cause later in life? What about the plastic baby bottles that have become so popular? What effect are they having on a growing infant? Remember that the effect of some of these chemicals, in the quantities we are exposed to, may not show any immediate or drastic symptoms. The problem may not show up until years have passed in a person's life.

I have already started eliminating plastics from my personal food chain. I have replaced plastic containers with glass ones, for any wet or liquid item. I still used plastic storage containers for dry products, but only when I haven't found the right glass storage container to replace them yet. One by one, I am getting rid of the plastic that comes in contact with food items.

You don't have to be fanatical in getting rid of plastics. Sometimes plastic containers are just more practical to use. It wouldn't be practical to send kids to school with a glass food container or glass pencil case. They would be heavy, and pose a possible injury risk if they broke.

Contact with the plastic can be mitigated by lining the container with wax paper or a paper towel. Stainless steel or aluminum containers are other options. They can be made very thin, and are lighter than glass would be. I have allocated many of the plastic containers I had on hand to storing physical items like cables, batteries, connectors, tools, and other non-food items.

2

Fats or Chemicals?

Is it the substitute fats or the chemical additives that are causing my weight problem? – I don't know. It could be one, the other, or a combination of the two. All I can suggest is that if you have a weight problem like mine, then as much as possible, stay away from products that contain these (and of course, do not use them at home). Governments around the world claim to be worried about the health of their citizens. But, as far as I know, no government is doing research into this particular problem, even though being overweight is connected to many health issues.

As long as an ingredient in a product is not obviously or immediately harmful to consumers, governments don't care that it is being sold to you. Subtle and long term effects never seem to come under scrutiny. In the United States, and some other countries, the definition of an "average" person has been changed to indicate that today it is a larger and heavier person than it was ten or twenty years ago (Gee! I wonder why?).

3

Product Advertisements

If you have been alive for a while, you will remember when

margarine was advertised as being the "healthier" alternative to butter (not true). Even today, substitute fats in one form or another are advertised as being the healthy choice. Younger people may not believe this, but there was a time when smoking was advertised as being good for your health (The government never stopped that, either). If, like myself, you are a coffee drinker, and you have been around for a while, you will recall hearing on news broadcasts that coffee was bad for you – only to be told some weeks later that coffee was good for you – again, to be told some time later that it was bad for you, etc., etc. GOOD – BAD – GOOD – BAD – and on, and on, and on again. This did not happen only for coffee. We have been given contradictory information about many foods and products, over the years. The only thing that I can tell you for certain is that, if the information is a product advertisement, you should be skeptical. No manufacturer is going to tell you that their product is bad for you. Nor are they going to tell you about any side effects unless there is a law that forces them to do so. When I say manufacturer, that includes makers of mass produced foods as well. Especially manufacturers of processed foods.

4

What it is that I do for myself

As I have stated before, I now stay away from mass produced baked goods. Sweets are my Achilles Heal, so I stay away from any mass produced sweet that I don't clearly know what it is made from. That doesn't mean all sweets that are mass produced need to be avoided. Also, the ingredients in sweets and treats are not the only reason to avoid them. You have to consider the calories as well.

As I have also stated before, the equation is relatively simple. If you take in more calories than your body uses up, you will likely gain weight. <u>The idea here is not to restrict your eating, but to start eating foods that are better for you, and made without questionable ingredients.</u> Foods that your body can utilize now, instead of storing it as fat for later use. But we have to face reality. In this modern world, we will be tempted by high calorie treats. To eliminate them completely would be beyond my personal self control (or desire).

As a practical compromise, I make most of my own treats, and I make them from scratch. That means that I know what all the ingredients are that go into them. I rarely use packaged mixes, even when the ingredients are clearly spelled out and they are not artificial or unknown to me. The result is that I am eating healthier, better-for-me foods that taste better, and I have a more varied diet. Yes, I do eat high calorie foods, and I do so often. But, my body now has reached a level of balance where my weight is not increasing.

I eat many delicious and varied items. Hungarian Goulash – yum. Sourdough and Herb biscuits – delicious. Banana, Chocolate Chip, Wheat Germ, or Cinnamon, etc. pancakes and waffles – absolutely! I have about a half-dozen different types of pancakes and waffles in my recipe book (which I eat with real butter and syrup, or fruit preserves to top them). Bacon-Jalapeno-and-Cheese cornbread – a tasty breakfast. Various types of cheesecakes – who doesn't love cheesecake???? Chicken and Pasta casserole, Shepard's pie, Meatloaf, Beef Stroganoff, various muffins and biscuits, Spanish Franks and Rice, Hamburgers with a side of Potato Salad, Pizza, Buttered Noodles (I think I could live on that), Chocolate Layer Cake, Carrot Cake (I love a good Carrot Cake), Pumpkin Roll with Cream Cheese icing, various types of cookies (of course). That's just a sampling of what I eat. You get the idea. My present day diet is definitely not restricted. It is in fact more varied than it was before.

Some readers might be thinking "That means I would have to cook. But, I don't know how to cook." or "I don't have time to cook." or "I don't want to cook." That is correct – sort of. Unless the lack of money is not a hindrance to you, you or someone you know would have to cook. I was lucky, in that I took a basic cooking course when I lived in the San Francisco Bay area, years ago (At the time, I didn't imagine how useful it would be). My culinary skills have greatly improved recently. I find cooking to be enjoyable – especially when I get to eat the results. I can make myself delicious foods that aren't available for sale locally. I like to try new recipes, and discovering new and delicious things to eat. Few things are as satisfying as making something that tastes delicious, and that you can make any time you want it. So, if you don't know how to cook, and don't have someone to cook for you, go out and sign up a cooking class at a local establishment. Go with some friends, and make it a social activity. The classes are both interesting and fun, and you get to eat what you make.

You really only have to learn the basic skills, and the meaning of some of the terminology. With just that, you should be able to follow a lot of recipes. If you don't think a cooking class is right for you, check out videos on the internet, where you can learn all kinds of skills while sitting at home (not to mention the plethora of step-by-step guided recipes available to you there).

5

Is there any help for the culinary inept?

You have probably seen the advertisements for meal kit service companies that will send you meal kits that include selected and portioned ingredients for each meal. There are many of those companies now. They do all the shopping for you, so that's a big help. However, you still have to cook the meals. As far as I can tell, it is all basic skill requirements, and since they come with instructions that should make it a little easier.

6

What else

I stay away from shortening, margarine, and any type of substitute ingredients, whenever I can. That doesn't mean I'm a fanatic about it. When I go to a restaurant, I have no idea of what they are cooking with (although sometimes you can taste it). For an occasional meal, it doesn't matter to me. If I ate every meal (or a lot of them) at restaurants, I would make it a point to find out what fats they are cooking with.

7

Artificial sweeteners – good or bad?

I do not know how the human body processes artificial sweeteners. I suspect they are not handled normally by the body, and may contribute to weight gain (just the opposite of what they are supposed to be for). But, that is just my personal opinion. They definitely fall into the "Processed" category, so I avoid them. I have tried some of them in different recipes and did not like the taste, so avoiding them is easy for me. Want another reason to avoid them? – they are expensive (and they taste bad). Their claim to fame is to have less calories than their sugar equivalent, but how can they be equivalent if they don't taste as good? What they should claim is that they are another (worse tasting) option, at best. If taste is your judgement criteria, artificial sweeteners can't be equivalent to natural sweeteners – in any quantity. Stick with the good stuff, the stuff that comes from nature and not from a laboratory.

Section 8

1

The local Boulangerie

If you like baked goods, and have a local bakery (a real bakery) nearby, treasure it and patronize it! By local bakery, I mean one that makes real food from real ingredients. I don't have a local bakery near me, I am sad to say. But when I travel, one of the first things I do is an internet search for one where I am staying. It has always been worth the effort.

Grocery store chains seem to all have bakery sections in them these days. I have talked to some of the people that work in them, and I have been told that some of the baked goods they sell are made from frozen, prepackaged dough. They have no idea what the ingredients in that dough are, and no reason to want to know (It's not their job). The chain's head office (in a galaxy far, far away) makes the decision of where to source the dough. The bakery section employees have no say-so about what is sent to them. Yes, some of it is baked on site – just not made on site. As is obvious when you walk their isles, a lot of the baked goods they sell come from commercial production facilities. The market reality is that if it is a product that people will buy, no retailer (none that I know of) is going to question what the ingredients are.

I was in a large chain store the other day. As I walked by the "bakery" section I came upon a table with stacks of boxed baked goods. It was quite a variety. I was going to just walk by it when I decided to take a look at some of the ingredients lists. The ingredients list for Chocolate Coconut Marble loaf cake had **45** ingredients listed!!!! 45 ingredients for a version of pound cake. Most of these ingredients (chemical additives) I have never heard of, and I certainly don't have them in my kitchen. Was I being too judgemental? When I got home, I did an internet search for recipes. I found several recipes for this type of cake, and the most complicated one had only 18 ingredients. The simplest one had 7 ingredients. Of these two examples of the cake, I had every ingredient in my kitchen, and I knew what each of them was. I looked at another item on the table. The ingredients list for Peanut Butter Fudge No Bake cookies had 17 ingredients. It's a simple cookie to make. I already make a similar cookie. It is very good, and one of my favorites (way too addictive). My recipe has only 7 ingredients. Yes, many of the ingredients listed on the commercial product were chemical additives.

What are these added chemicals doing to our bodies? Especially, what are they doing to my body, and the bodies of those people with the same weight problem I have? The answer is that no one knows. No one that I have heard of has looked into this. There is another problem with these mass produced "baked goods", and that is they don't taste very good compared to when made with natural ingredients.

2

If I want to try this concept, what should I do?

I will try to itemize what needs to be done, but you have to remember that people have such varied eating habits that I cannot cover everything in a list. Another problem is that I don't have a defined list of what additives are causing the weight gain problem. This is something that should be investigated by medical professionals and researchers. But, here goes:

- Do not eat any cookies or baked goods that are mass produced if the ingredient list has chemicals or items that you are not familiar with (defined as not found in the average home kitchen). If you are not familiar with common baking ingredients, ask someone who is. If you buy these from a local chain "bakery" or an actual bakery, ask for an ingredient list or stop buying from them. Remember that not all ingredients may appear on the list. Tell them your concerns, and that you are avoiding chemical additives.

- Processed foods that follow the previous "don't eat" criteria should also be off your list. Remember, there is a difference between "processed" and "frozen" or "canned". Again, check the ingredients. Some frozen or canned foods have also been chemically processed and contain ingredients that you might want to avoid. Others don't have these additives. Check the label.

- Canned foods (in cans or bottles) also need to be scrutinized. Check the ingredients list. If it is just a can that is mainly of a few known ingredients (canned beans, tuna, vegetables, etc.) it is probably alright. If you see those strange and unpronounceable names in the ingredients list, don't buy them. I will state again, that if you are not sure, you can try it and see what effect it has on you, but that procedure is only helpful after you have stabilized your weight.

- Remember that not all ingredients are always listed. Sometimes the only way to know if a product is acceptable is to try it. Unless you know where every item in your diet comes from, you cannot get away from chemical processing completely. It wouldn't be practical, and may not be necessary. Not all of the chemicals with strange names may be causing your weight problem. But, who wants to eat chemicals anyway? You want to get as much of them out of your diet as you can.

- When it comes to meals, either make your own or buy from a place that you know doesn't use chemically processed ingredients in their food. If there is any doubt, ask them if they do. Restaurant managers I have talked to have had no problem telling me what their ingredients are, and most very proudly tell me they do not use any processed items.

- You cannot be one hundred percent sure all the time, as to which foods are good for you and which aren't. You don't have to be a fanatic about this. Take it slow and easy as you scrutinize which foods are acceptable. Eating the wrong food occasionally will probably not hurt your effort. I do it every now and then. Sometimes it is unavoidable.

- Eat REAL food and use REAL ingredients, and not substitutes. Use real butter, lard, bacon grease, olive oil, or vegetable oil, etc., in your cooking and baking. Don't throw away that delicious bacon grease. Save it to fry your foods in. What? – You don't consider bacon grease as being healthy? Then use real olive oil or another vegetable oil to fry in. It's really your choice. To put it simply, use natural fats in your diet. I would stay away from margarines and shortenings as much as possible.

Sweeten with sugar, honey, maple syrup, or other natural sweeteners, and not artificial sweeteners. Personally, I have tried artificial sweeteners throughout the years and haven't found one that I like the taste of. To summarize – Go all natural as much as you can.

3

I have stabilized my weight, but

now want to lose some

If you are getting the same results as I have (hopefully, even a little better), and are eating more calories (spelled S-W-E-E-T-S for me) while remaining stable, you should be able to lose some weight by cutting back slightly on the treats. By slightly, I mean to a point where you are not having cravings or feeling deprived. You can also increase your physical activity which will utilize more of the calories you have taken in. Doing this should cause some weight loss, but at a very slow rate. If your intent is to lose tens of pounds in a few months, then going to a weight LOSS program is probably your best bet. After you have lost the weight you can get back on the stabilization concept to prevent weight gain. Personally, I can only stay on a weight loss program for a few months at the longest. I will probably do just that sometime in the future, but right now I am still experimenting with the stabilization concept. Pushing the limits a little to learn how I am affected, and by what.

4

WOW! You've read all the way through the book.

If you have read this far through the book, then by now you know that this concept – this "diet" – really has nothing to do with chocolate chip cookies, or eating other sweets and treats. What it is really about is **the foods you select to eat, the additives that have been put in them, and the unknown effects they have on us**. Understanding these detrimental effects is the first step. I do not know how many people are being affected weight wise by these additives. I don't know of any research that has been done on the subject. Body weight may not be, and probably isn't, the only thing being affected by these additives. It is just the obvious one. I wonder what else these chemicals are doing to our bodies in a way that is so subtle that we are not aware of it. What serious damage is being caused, that doesn't show up for years, and is not being associated with the ingestion (or exposure by other means) of these chemicals? Consider that these chemicals are going into our bodies in low doses (No immediate and obvious adverse reaction to them) over a long period of time. They are deemed safe to use in our food because they are not killing lab rats when used in relatively large quantities over a short period of time. The truth is that we are the real lab rats, in an experiment that, as far as I know, no one is monitoring. It is left completely up to us as individuals to find out how this is affecting us. What damage (injury) is being done to our bodies, that can't be reversed?

I wish I had the facilities to record the results of everyone that tries this concept, so that we could all see what is going on. As

48

far as I know, and as of this writing, I am the only person documenting this concept and its effect on my body weight. I urge you to keep a record of your results. Below is a simple spreadsheet format that you can follow. Modify it as you like. It will give you an idea of the most basic elements of your diet to record. You can do this on a computer or a piece of paper. Expand on it if you wish. More data can only be more useful.

I hope that this concept helps as many people as possible. I wish everyone who tries it, improving health, and the very best of health throughout their lives.

ADDENDUM

1

Basic Spreadsheet

You can keep track of your results by logging the DATE, WEIGHT, and EXTRA STUFF I ATE THIS WEEK information. Do it on a computer spreadsheet or a piece of paper. Keep track of other items if it suits you to do so. It is important to keep track of these items so that you can see if the stabilization concept is working for you, and what food items may be affecting you badly.

2

As promised – My personal record

Below is a copy of the actual spreadsheet I have been tracking my weight with, and below that is a chart derived from that data. It is up to date as of the date of this publication. What is important to note are the weight readings over time, and all the **extra** treats I ate during each week. This does not show the regular meals or any of my standby chocolate chip cookies that I have eaten throughout that week. For those curious about it, I usually make and eat at least one batch of those cookies (18 – 20 two inch cookies) per week, and sometimes more than that. Any items listed in the chart below are in addition to that. Where no quantities are given, it means I had consumed the complete container or batch of what is listed in the week previous to my weigh-in – i.e., Where ice cream is mentioned without a quantity it means I ate the whole 1.5 quarts – the whole standard size container it is sold in, during that previous week. Where a cake or pie is listed without a quantity it means I ate the whole cake or pie (in that previous week).

You will notice some discrepancies at the beginning dates of my weight tracking. This was at a time when I was just beginning to realize what was going on, and had not yet decided to track it on a regular basis. It was around the middle of March of 2021 that I began weekly measurements.

DATE	WEIGHT	EXTRAS
11-13-2020	193.8	
12-17-2020	192.4	
1-08-2021	192.2	
1-15-2021	192.2	
1-20-2021	192.2	
1-30-2021	190.6	
2-07-2021	191.2	
3-02-2021	194.0	4 packages of chocolate covered pretzels
3-06-2021	192.2	
3-13-2021	192.8	
3-20-2021	190.8	
3-27-2021	191.0	box of chocolate mini-donuts from Walmart
4-03-2021	191.8	French Chocolate Gateaux Baulois this week
4-10-2021	192.0	7 chocolate covered peanut bars
4-13-2021	190.8	
4-17-2021	191.4	9 chocolate covered peanut bars.
4-24-2021	190.6	5 slices cheese cake
5-01-2021	190.6	9 Oatmeal Chocolate Peanut Butter Cookies this past Sunday. Had a few slices of cheese cake this week.
5-08-2021	190.8	pan of cornmeal brownies
5-15-2021	190.1	Pan of cornmeal brownies & Choco-Peanut Butter ice cream
5-22-2021	190.6	Chocolate-peanut butter bars & Choco-Peanut Butter ice cream
5-29-2021	191.2	Cadbury milk chocolate bar, Choco-Peanut Butter Ice cream
6-05-2021	190.2	Baker's Semi Sweet baking chocolate bar
6-12-2021	192.0	Choco-Peanut Butter ice cream, oatmeal chocolate peanut butter cookies
6-19-2021	190.6	Carrot cake with Cream Cheese icing, 2/3 Cadbury milk chocolate bar
6-26-2021	192.0	Baker's Semi-sweet chocolate bar and 1 liter Chocolate Peanut Butter Cup ice cream
7-3-2021	192.4	Loaf of pumpkin bread, chocolate-peanut butter ice cream.
7-10-2021	192.8	batch of brownies, chocolate-peanut butter ice cream.
7-17-2021	192.4	4 blueberry muffins with streusel topping, various nuts, chocolate chips, graham crackers
7-24-2021	192.4	Halva, chocolate-peanut butter ice cream., 4 blueberry muffins with streusel topping
7-31-2021	191.0	Cadbury milk chocolate bar, 4 slices Chocolate Cloud Pie
8-7-2021	191.6	2 slices Chocolate Cloud pie, chocolate-peanut butter ice cream., 6 raspberry muffins
8-14-2021	190.0	loaf of banana bread, large milk chocolate candy bar
8-21-2021	190.4	Loaf of chocolate banana bread, 1 liter choco-peanut butter ice cream.

Notice on the chart below how my weight measurements jump up and down. This is why weighing yourself only once a week and looking at the trend is the only useful way to track your results.

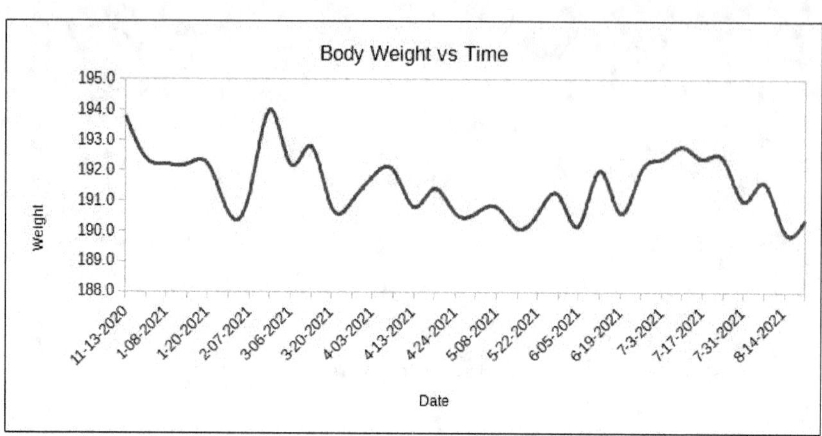

Body Weight vs Time
Weight
195.0
194.0
193.0
192.0
191.0
190.0
189.0
188.0
11-13-2020
1-08-2021
1-20-2021
2-07-2021
3-06-2021
3-20-2021
4-03-2021
4-13-2021
4-24-2021
5-08-2021
5-22-2021
6-05-2021
6-19-2021
7-3-2021
7-17-2021
7-31-2021
8-14-2021
Date